Table of Contents

Comprehensive Overview of Acute Liver Failure

1. Introduction to Acute Liver Failure

1.1. Definition and Epidemiology

1.2. Types of Liver Failure

2. Symptoms of Acute Liver Failure

2.1. Common Symptoms

2.2. Less Common Symptoms

3. Causes of Acute Liver Failure

3.1. Viral Infections

3.2. Drug-Induced Liver Injury

3.3. Autoimmune Hepatitis

4. Diagnosis of Acute Liver Failure

4.1. Clinical Evaluation

4.2. Laboratory Tests

4.3. Imaging Studies

5. Treatment of Acute Liver Failure

5.1. Supportive Care

5.2. Liver Transplantation

5.3. Specific Treatments for Underlying Causes

Comprehensive Study on Acute Liver Failure Caused by Acetaminophen Overdose

1. Introduction to Acute Liver Failure

1.1. Definition and Classification

1.2. Epidemiology and Incidence

2. Pathophysiology of Acute Liver Failure

2.1. Normal Liver Function

2.2. Mechanism of Acetaminophen Toxicity

3. Clinical Presentation

3.1. Symptoms and Signs

3.2. Diagnostic Evaluation

4. Management of Acute Liver Failure

4.1. General Supportive Care

4.2. Specific Treatment Options

5. Prognosis and Complications

5.1. Factors Affecting Prognosis

5.2. Potential Complications

6. Prevention Strategies

6.1. Public Health Interventions

6.2. Patient Education

7. Conclusion and Future Directions

Comprehensive Overview of Acute Liver Failure

1. Introduction to Acute Liver Failure

1.1. Definition and Epidemiology

1.2. Types of Liver Failure

2. Symptoms of Acute Liver Failure

Clinical consequences of acute liver injury are paradoxically a result of both decreased and increased hepatic functions. Most patients complain of viral-like symptoms like weakness, myalgia, and signs of jaundice. Nausea and vomiting are also reported, alongside other symptoms like fever, arthralgia, or rash. In severe paracetamol toxicity, symptoms may often appear after a latency phase of almost 24 hours. The half-life of paracetamol excretion is prolonged in older individuals, which might result in a somewhat later manifestation of the injury. Pharmaceutical compounds and bacteria can accumulate during the progression of severe hepatic necrosis. Permanent hepatic disorder ensues when neutrophils, lymphocytes, or foreign-body giant cells bind to these noxious agents. Viruses with direct cytopathogenicity produce local inflammation when specific immunopathogenic cells, macrophages, and Kupffer cells are recruited. Even though viral hepatitis is caused by the triad, the condition is self-limited or reactive. Unscheduled beta-oxidation during short-term paracetamol therapy results in potential quinoneimine-induced decompression of hepatic swelling. Aminotransferases are astonishingly elevated with granulocyte infiltration. Oxford criteria relate to the initial stages of hepatic encephalopathy when treating acute liver failure: the onset of coagulopathy, synthesized hepatic encephalopathy or altered consciousness with hepatic encephalopathy grade III-IV leads to suspicion of hypoglycemia as a rare alternative neurotoxic criterion. An unclear confounding diagnosis or an interval to encephalopathy of fewer than 7 days is taken into account in the diagnosis. Data gathered appear to suggest that patients with infectious hepatitis with grade I toxicity of metavir on histology may pass hepatic encephalopathy grade III-IV.

SYMPTOMS

An immense challenge faced by clinicians arises from the complexity of severe liver injury. Nearly 500,000 people every year are inflicted by acute liver failure. This condition arises concomitantly with the absence of any pre-existing known liver disease in the populace. A manifold increase in the rate of this dangerous disease has been reported. Acute liver failure results in rapid deterioration of hepatocellular function, presented clinically by severe coagulopathy and encephalopathy and severe disruption in metabolism. It has been widely held that hyperacute submassive necrosis is the harrowing leading cause of severe liver dysfunctions, as noted in liver biopsies or necropsies of nearly all instances of severe liver destruction. Hepatitis A and B viruses, drugs and toxins, ischemic insults, and paracetamol poisoning are the leading causes of severe liver injury. In an attempt to shift the hepatic pathophysiology towards normal, liver transplantation serves as a method for patients suffering from acute liver failure, but lack of donor organs can impede the process. Acute liver failure results from sudden loss of functional hepatocytes, concomitant with hepatic encephalopathy and coagulopathy in patients without previously known liver disease. Acute liver failure is a clinical syndrome, characterized by direct damage to the liver leading to elevated aminotransferases: aspartate aminotransferase, alanine aminotransferase. It is difficult to recognize the clinical signs and symptoms of hepatic deterioration in the very young, old, or when pronounced hepatocyte destruction precedes the loss of hepatic functions, acute liver failure prevails. Hyperacute submassive necrosis happens to be the primary cause of rapid liver dysfunction in the population. Apart from that, two neighboring minute compartments exist in hepatic sinusoids, Disse spaces, in mixed alcoholic liver degeneration, improved density of Kupffer as well as Ito cells, and in hepatitis B for continuous coagulation necrosis.

2.1. Common Symptoms

Patients with acute liver failure may develop fever and/or an ileus in the absence of infection. Pulmonary, cardiovascular, and renal manifestations are common. Pulmonary complications may include acute respiratory distress syndrome and pulmonary edema. At the cardiovascular level, hypotension, hypertension, and arrhythmias are seen. At the renal level, acute kidney injury is often observed. The underlying etiologies may be broadly categorized as infectious, ischemic, immunologic, or toxin-related. The main symptoms of acute liver failure include parenchymal hepatocellular damage (jaundice, encephalopathy, hepatic biochemical dysfunction), a reduction in hepatic detoxification (coagulopathy, elevation of serum ammonia, hypoglycemia), and all other unrelated systemic failures (renal-dialysis, pulmonary, cardiovascular, hematology).

The patient may present with bile duct disease, encephalopathy, hyperbilirubinemia (i.e., serum bilirubin $\geq$ 15 mg/dL), lactic acidosis (i.e., serum lactate $\geq$ 1.5 mmol/L), coagulopathy (i.e., INR $\geq$ 1.5), and progressive ascites (i.e., the patient not identified to have hepatic encephalopathy on examination). The rapidity of the progression to hepatic encephalopathy is a hallmark of acute liver failure. Because of encephalopathy, patients may have asterixis. Additionally, the patient may have a very tender and enlarged liver, and confusion, but not marked weakness or jaundice. Patients with acute liver failure often develop cerebral edema and an increase in intracranial pressure.

2.2. Less Common Symptoms

Most patients who develop acute liver failure already have known symptoms. Occasionally, acute liver failure symptoms arise before obvious jaundice. Periodic nausea and fatigue are not uncommon but are often overlooked as the possible heralding symptoms of disease. Therefore, their presence has more significance than their absence. Vomiting, whether bilious or of red blood from bleeding of esophageal varices, can be an early symptom of liver disease. It is frequently intractable between presumed flu episodes or stomach viral infection attacks. Retinal bleeding (retinopathy) may be hallmarks of acute liver failure in the pediatric population. Patients may also develop weight loss. If the patient is not suffering from viral hepatitis "E" and "C", alterations in taste and anorexia are unusual. Because of the limited intact normal liver mass, patients develop ascites or lower extremity edema relatively late compared to chronic liver disease.

Mental status alteration might be an atypical presentation of acute liver failure in up to 50% of patients. Impaired judgment, disinhibition, marked mood or personality change, or lethargy might occur prior to the less commonly associated vomiting with blood or collapsing from loss of blood or even jaundice. Hallucinations, whether visual, auditory, or olfactory, have been reported. Unexplained bruising (ecchymosis on multiple body areas), spontaneous nosebleeds (epistaxis), unusual or multiple petechiae, or inflammatory pustules from hair follicles (folliculitis) on the face and neck regions may occur before the more recognizable coagulopathy.

Less common (atypical) symptoms of acute liver failure

3. Causes of Acute Liver Failure

Several factors may cause acute liver injuries: ischaemia (1) and toxic liver diseases. In resource-rich countries, most viral hepatitis, Epstein-Barr, and cytomegalovirus account for almost 70% of patients beyond age 10 and nearly 30% of the remaining patients unexpectedly involving unknown causes. In children, 40-70% of cases are due to drug overdoses, hepatitis, Amanita mushroom poisoning, and other drugs. In children, approximately 25% of cases are indeterminate. Bacterial endotoxinaemia as one factor may have a key role. Predicting non-B non-G infectious recoveries depends critically on an improved understanding of endetteataneous associations or hyperimmunity. Other drugs such as ecstasy, ephedrine, ephedrine (such as those used to treat coughs and colds, V. parahaemolyticus or mycobacteria such as the NTM of cholangiohepatitis, Histoplasma, as well as drugs such as aripiprazole, bipolar disorder, and fasuloth are worth banishing whatever their guises. (2) Potential cannabinoids (Cannabis sativa renum/) used to treat chronic pain, fibromyalgia, and multiple sclerosis as pill Marinol/Dronabinol or vaporizer extract may be relevant to the pro- or anti-NAFLD and NASH reader. (3) Acetaminophen-induced acute liver failure's (AALF) (AAP) cytosolic metabolite N-acetyl-p-benzocin-quonointments release HASMD and HASWI to degrade eeG or it exploit GT1-CH genes and other Z-virus to mediate their spread throughout organisms and ecosystems locally, regionally, or nationally—or the world. Such pre-C storage tend to act a list in so-called blowback. (4) Iatrogenic (infiltrationism) acute liver failure may stem from such manifold category of malpractices as wound dehiscence. Ear, nose and throat consultations, maxillofacial schotoma, rhinoplasty, facelift, and skin grafts are all trendy, whether these women or men are overtly foolish or secretly scorned vessels. (5) Selective brain exhaustion of sulfite (increased in the sea) with direct entry of a newly USA-patent-approved (#5,500,647/9,454,236) marketable, under-the-table, non-prescription nutritional snack food, brown-to-red acid hydrolysates of reconstituted tomatoes dissolved in sulfite/bisulfite/metabisulfite-allowed (permitted) endo-vitamin consumption into the hepatic portal vein from the gastrointestinal tract.

In general, acute liver failure can be triggered through: direct hepatocyte injury (taking paracetamol/acetaminophen, viral hepatitis), injury to the microvasculature (bacterial endotoxin or endogenous/endotoxins), immune reaction against hepatocytes (ischemia and reperfusion injury), or injury to mitochondria leading to apoptosis or necrosis (drug like cocaine or agent like Amanita) or oxidative stress (Reye's syndrome). Specific causes include the following, amongst others: drug, toxins, such as mushrooms, viruses such as hepatitis A, B or E, or drugs such as liver failure or paracetamol (acetaminophen or APAP) or ibuprofen or NSAIDs, or overdose of OTC-pharmacotherapeutics, sickness to Wilson's illness or Wilson's diseases and jaundice or infections to Herpes simplex virus and infected or influenza or idiopathic or anaphylaxis.

3.1. Viral Infections

Viral agents in general are considered to stimulate the immune system cells during the infection period, leading to T cells reactive to the expression of these antigens on the hepatocytes. This stimulated immune system subsets subsequently kill specifically virus-infected hepatocytes which present these antigens on their cells. This cellular immune attack consequently destroys a considerable number of normal hepatic cells as well as the virus-infected cells, as they have hepatocytes belonging to the same non-specific target. Infection in the initial phase and unfavorable factors in the immune system cause a loss in liver replacement potential - Kupffer cells are the main cause of necrotic necrosis in acute liver failure (ALF). It has been highlighted that Kupffer cells usually show more severe hyperfunction in fulminant hepatitis and the destruction of liver entry and exit bilirubin cells increases the level of bilirubin more frequently. Kupffer cell hyperactivation weakens endothelial energy via oncotic mediator liberation recruiting more neutrophil leukocytes involving in endothelial veranda. Kupffer cell depletion and closure can also exacerbate the inflammatory response.

Viral infections are the most common etiological factors in the pathogenesis of acute liver failure. Viruses are found to trigger the process of acute liver failure and lead to severe damage in a short period of time. Based on the data recorded between different case series, 3-7 children in every 100 with viral hepatitis developed severe fulminant hepatic failure. HBV, HAV, HDV, HEV, HCV and Parvovirus

B-19 infections are some viral etiological factors that may cause acute liver failure. Children who have developed fulminant hepatitis B (hepatitis B symptoms are observed in more than 90%) account for 4% of all HBV infections in children. Perinatal infection, when infected with hepatitis B, increases the risk of developing fulminant hepatitis, and fulminant hepatitis is seen in 20% of infected babies during the neonatal period. The clinical spectrum can range from subclinical to jaundice in the clinical presentation of hepatitis, especially in HDV infections, but fast progression and severe fulminant acute liver failure can be seen as in hepatitis Delta co-infections.

3.2. Drug-Induced Liver Injury

Most cases of acute liver failure are due to paracetamol [acetaminophen] overdose. When an overdose or a specific non-overdose is taken, the metabolic pathways that do not detoxify the reactive intermediates are conjugated to glutathione (GSH), and other sulfur-containing compounds are converted by different isoenzymes of the P-450 monooxygenase and cytochrome system in the liver. When the starting amount of the toxic intermediate is more, or the available GSH stores are depleted, these enzyme systems become overwhelmed within a period and this generally happens within 12-19 h. This leads to the subsequent production of the covalently bound complex between the intermediate and the cytochrome P-450 system, currently believed to be an important mechanism of 'mitochondrial damage'. At the same time, profound hepatic centrilobular [zone 3] necrosis also occurs due to the toxic intermediates (N-acetyl-p-benzo-quinoneimines) which develop in the cytoplasm. The clinical features that have been released in the recent period are universally agreed upon. In the UK, patients may now only be offered intensive care and a liver transplant (very rarely an auxiliary liver at the time of writing) if they develop stage 3 encephalopathy (hepatic), because of the excellent and supportive care in the ICU and liver units they receive.

A considerable number of pharmacological agents and different medications or drugs are used for their immunosuppressant qualities in the patients receiving liver transplant, as well as in the intensive care unit. Many available medications in the field of supportive ICU care, individual drugs being the major cause of acute liver failure. Their impact depends on many factors such as chronic liver disease, age, and genetic makeup of the individual patients among others. The other medications include valproic acid, carbamazepine, and antiretroviral agents. Arsenic and Amanita toxins can also be the causes of acute liver failure.

3.3. Autoimmune Hepatitis

It has not been definitively clarified yet whether the organ-specific LKM1- or LKM2-reactive T-cells and B-cells originate in the liver or in lesions of other organs modified intracellularly in the same way as the previously tolerized LKM1- and LKM2-antigens. The phenomenon is reminiscent of the reactions of T-cells in hepatitis C and D in which cross-reactions in other intracellularly modified cells also seem to cause disease. These data are based on comparative investigations of organ-specific T-cells in blood samples and bone marrow biopsies. In general, the leukocyte populations in the liver and in the blood do not differ at least in patients with type 1 autoimmune hepatitis. Currently, the rejection of tolerogenic pathways of the immune system and the resulting side effects predominate as a result of an interruption in treatment with primary prophylaxis.

Autoimmune mechanisms do not play an important role in the development of ALF and hyperacute liver failure alone, but they can often lead to a poor prognosis. The onset of ALF is usually accompanied by additional immune responses in the liver. In most patients, signs of the activation of complement components and the production of antibodies in the blood against components of the liver, for instance, LKM1 (liver and kidney microsomes 1), are present. LKM1-antibodies IgG are autoantibodies against cytochrome P450, and their presence enables the diagnosis of AIH type 2. In a collective with more than 300 adult patients, 9% of the patients showed an increased anti-

LKM2 IgG level. This had no influence on survival, although slightly more patients required liver transplantation.

4. Diagnosis of Acute Liver Failure

Diagnosis is from medical history: The diagnosis of acute liver failure is made from the medical history and is a clinical diagnosis. No serologic test results are required for diagnosis; on presentation of hepatic failure in a previously healthy individual, immediate patient evaluation and investigation are ordered. If serologic tests are required for specific etiologies (e.g., Wilson's disease or autoimmune hepatitis), the patient is diagnosed with fulminant hepatic failure if the rapid onset of jaundice that is the hallmark of active liver disease is present. Testing for acetaminophen overdose is often done in the United States in accordance with the key clinical feature of accidental overdose or young suicidal behavior. Early diagnosis and rapid prioritization are the primary objectives of management of acute liver failure because of the seriousness of the clinical disease, and serologic tests are not specific or sensitive in this condition.

In a patient presenting to the clinic with altered mental status or sudden onset jaundice in an otherwise previously healthy individual, the diagnosis of acute liver failure is made from the medical history. Acute liver failure is a clinical diagnosis made when a previously healthy individual presents with severe hepatic failure as evidenced by altered mental status and coagulopathy. Acute liver failure is also called fulminant liver failure in some countries in association with deteriorating liver function. Chronic liver failure is a separate condition that results from long-term malnutrition or cirrhosis. The previous healthy status of acute liver failure patients differentiates the condition from other newer, more chronic forms of liver failure and necessitates rapid patient management without a long organ sickness waiting list and prioritization system. In the majority of patients, liver transplantation is the most effective therapy for acute liver failure.

4.1. Clinical Evaluation

It was reported that a large proportion of patients underwent liver biopsy to establish the diagnosis. Liver biopsy can also produce negative results that delay appropriate management and may be painful, though the ALFSG LLRs have made it possible for clinicians to stratify patients with a low probability of benefiting from bedside biopsy of the liver. Extensive experience indicates that significant hemorrhage related to liver biopsy is rare and, even in the presence of a coagulopathy, biopsy can be performed with an adequate safety margin. Expert biopsy supervision is advisable in the presence of coagulopathy, however, given that the transjugular approach may be associated with lower morbidity. A complete blood count and other hematologic parameters (international normalized ratio, partial thromboplastin time, and platelet count) always need to be determined before the performance of a liver biopsy, and these parameters should be reviewed for the target study. Diniz et al. explained that "[s]everal patients with ALF are hypercoagulable and, as a result, could develop thrombosis at the site of percutaneous biopsy. Additionally, because of associated coagulopathy, patients with cirrhosis and ACLF have shown a higher risk of bleeding after percutaneous liver biopsy." Likewise, in patients with contraindications to transjugular biopsy, ultrasound guidance may enable a safe and reliable technique to be employed. While Dixit et al. documented microcoagulation in the liver biopsy of a patient using the transjugular technique, the generally lower morbidity and hemorrhagic risk of transjugular biopsy means that this technique is advisable in patients with thrombocytopenia or coagulopathies. Biopsies can be carried out under splenorenal angiographic pressure conditions, and an internal shunt insertion may permit biopsy while the patient is under general anesthesia. Biopsy decides more than one etiology in 30% of cases and is, thus, a useful diagnostic tool. However, depending on the patient's clinical status, the presence of multiple advanced disease etiologies rather than a single underlying process is a contraindication to transplantation. Biopsy should not be performed in critically ill patients who are not considered candidates for liver transplantation.

After taking the history and physical examination, the evaluation of patients with suspected ALF includes specific tests to establish the diagnosis and determine the etiology. Although liver biopsy can be a valuable tool in establishing the etiology of suspected ALF, it is generally not required, as important prognostic information can often be obtained from a combination of the clinical history, imaging studies, and selected laboratory tests (i.e., acetaminophen/paracetamol and salicylate levels, viral serologies, and toxin screens for nonviral agents such as amanita phalloides). In a cross-sectional analysis of patients with ALF performed contemporaneously with enrollment in the ALF Study, however, the wide variability in presentation of ALF etiologies and the potential for rare and previously undiagnosed conditions.

4.2.2. Hematological Investigations Hemoglobin percentage, red blood cell count, hematocrit levels, erythrocyte sedimentation rate, and white blood cell count are assessed to screen diffuse or focal inflammatory processes in the patient along with the accompanying appropriate symptoms like fever, chills, and cough. The male and female routine hematology reference intervals provide guidance at presentation for diagnoses, treatment, risk stratification, clinical follow-up, and compliance with transfusion thresholds in acute conditions.

4.2.1. Biochemical Analyses Liver function tests are conducted to verify the presence of hepatic synthetic functions. Serum albumin, bilirubin, and the prothrombin time are interpreted as synthetic functions of the liver. Low albumin and increased bilirubin levels are mostly attributable to chronic liver disease. White blood cells and differential values are done to look for acute or chronic infections. Urea, creatinine, and electrolytes are assessed to look into hepato-renal malfunctions in the body. Venous blood gas analysis is performed to check acidosis and its cause. A serum lactate level by way of a single measurement has no marked value in acute liver failure patients. The elevated blood lactate level indicates an anaerobic metabolism, which is an indicator of hypoperfusion, hypoxemia, or a combination of both. Pure L-lactic acidosis (metabolic lactic acidosis) is an early sign of liver failure.

A meticulous diagnostic workup is crucial for acute liver failure, and therefore, diagnosis is often possible through clinical and biochemical means. The initial laboratory test is an attempt to diagnose an underlying cause, prognosticate patients, and rule out acute liver failure mimickers.

4.3. Imaging Studies

Since ALF is a clinical syndrome that typically occurs in patients without any known previous liver disease, no radiologic or other imaging techniques are needed to confirm the diagnosis. However, radiologic examinations play a role in ALF patients by showing the causes of admission and demonstrating complications and collateral effects. Positions of technicians or radiologists, advantages, and disadvantages of the imaging technique used or technique proposed for new liver acquisitions should be stated. The techniques suggested might not differentiate between causes of ALF but identify or confirm reduced liver volume and function versus normal liver volume and function.

Imaging techniques play an important role in determining the etiology of acute liver failure (ALF) by demonstrating the underlying pathological condition and allowing evaluation of diminished hepatic structure and/or function. Although grey-scale US, CT, MRI, or hybrid techniques are employed, to date, no guideline suggests using any of those techniques as the preferred choice. Colour Doppler US, dynamic and perfusion CT, hepatocellular-specific MRI, MRI elastography, and CT/MRI HAP scoring sequences are more advanced imaging techniques that may be useful when the diagnosis has to be confirmed or excluded in combination with clinical data, laboratory tests, and liver histopathology. GB US, CEUS, bile-duct MRI, and MRCP are primary imaging modalities to identify GB stones and are particularly useful when in doubt, with CT/MRI HAP scoring sequences and hepatic volumetries being also important when a real volume deficit has to be demonstrated or quantified.

5. Treatment of Acute Liver Failure

In summary, acute liver failure is a dramatic syndrome, defined by coagulopathy (INR > 1.5) and hepatic encephalopathy, frequently complicated by cerebral edema due to increased brain water content. The prospect of an effective medical treatment based on an understanding of the cellular and molecular mechanisms of brain edema using less invasive procedures such as microdialysis awaits further research on crucial pathophysiologic issues in animal models and human biopsies. In the meantime, liver transplantation remains an option to save the life of a patient with severe acute liver failure who is not improving after optimal supportive treatment. However, recent data suggest that the demand for liver transplantation in acute liver failure may be decreasing, possibly due to an increased efficacy of supportive treatment and hope of the development of new guidelines on liver transplantation for severe acute liver failure in the near future, including secondary transplantation and the problem of high urgency listing. Predictive scores will help make such guidelines more reliable and consistent.

Prevention of intracranial hypertension is primarily managed with elevating the head, intubation with hyperventilation to maintain a pCO_2 of 30-35 mm Hg (4-4.7 kPa), and using an osmotic agent: 20% mannitol or 50% hypertonic saline. Albumin infusions are indicated when plasma albumin levels are low. Gastrointestinal bleeding should also be excluded using endoscopy. Because of the potential infection-related intracranial hypertension following liver transplantation, patients should never be screened for infection until they are actually symptomatic or febrile. Only a biopsy can provide a definitive diagnosis of liver damage.

5.1. Supportive Care

If necessary, they should take low doses of calcium supplements. If albumin drops below 20 g/L, a dose of 20% albumin at 1 g/kg LW should be infused daily until albumin rises to a value of over 25 g/L.

Central to the care of patients with ALF is maintaining effective nutrition and hydroelectrolytic balance using an accurate, heavily protein-based solution combined with a restricted sodium content to be carried out in a suitable setting and by a skilled healthcare team. It is also crucial that a vigilant system of care is in place to maintain these patients' nutritional and fluid equilibrium, since these are often the primary candidate for urgent LT in cases of ALF. The patient's volume of intravenous fluids is substituted on a daily basis at less than 1000 mL/day of enteral feeding.

Care should be conducted in an intensive or high-dependency setting with ongoing assessment of the airway, breathing, and circulation. The management of ALF includes measurement of the temperature, white cell count, nutritional considerations (including the prevention of hypoglycemia and rarely of nasojejunal enteral nutrition to avoid protein catabolism), and a careful diagnostic workup. Monitoring temperature, pulse, mean arterial pressure, urinary output, oxygen saturation, close observation of the neurological state, or Glasgow Coma Scale (GCS), and serial blood lactate concentrations are the most clinically important parameters.

The cornerstone of treatment in ALF is supportive measures. Stabilizing and maintaining the patient is the major focus of therapy with or without LT. The goal of care is to maintain the vital signs, prevent and treat complications, and manage OHCs. Interventions need to occur as early as possible to prevent secondary injury to the liver.

5.1. Supportive Care

5.2. Liver Transplantation

Healthy patients with ALF and "unlimited" MELD scores should not be considered for livers from older deceased donors, because such livers are critically ill upon transplantation. Hepatitis A is generally the best indication for liver transplantation in patients who are hemodynamically stable, as the donor liver is not infected and antiviral therapy is available to prevent reinfection post-TX. It appears reasonable not to actively list patients with drug-induced ALF for liver transplantation if they are not observed to improve rapidly after the withdrawal of the implicated drug or drugs. However, the liver can unexpectedly recover during the first few days of treatment, and in the absence of a medical judgment the case should therefore be discussed in a multidisciplinary team meeting. Providing a structured workup is performed, an initial removal of a patient from the waiting list for liver transplantation does not affect the chances of survival with a native liver compared to continuing to remain on the waiting list.

Liver transplantation: Orthotopic liver transplantation is currently the only life-saving therapeutic option for patients with ALF, and is usually futile outside of liver transplantation centres. Improved outcomes after liver transplantation for ALF have paralleled improvements in perioperative care and perioperative treatment for intracranial hypertension and for prevention and treatment of systemic inflammatory response syndrome. As patients with ALF fulfill standard criteria for prioritizing patients for liver transplantation, the outcome for patients with ALF treated with liver transplantation is the same as for patients transplanted for other indications, with 1-year survival after liver transplantation in patients transplanted for ALF of around 85%. Super-urgent allocation of a liver graft to a patient with ALF outside of the usual priority system is unnecessary unless the patient also has a chronic history of liver disease that fulfilled super-urgent criteria for transplantation before the onset of ALF.

5.3. Specific Treatments for Underlying Causes

The only disease-specific intervention in acetaminophen-induced acute liver failure is the antidote treatment N-acetylcysteine (NAC). Acetylcysteine - the adapted antidote regime for acetaminophen poisoning is able to effectively bind the hepatotoxic acetaminophen adduct (NAPQI) in plasma. The administration of N-acetylcysteine is effective only when the first dose (oral or intravenous) is administered early, ideally in an outpatient setting or emergency room less than 8 hours after ingestion and certainly within 16 hours. NAC should be continued until the clinical improvement of the patient, which occurs once available hepatic glutathione captures and detoxifies sufficient NAPQI. Oral administration of immediate release NAC is recommended. If there is no clinical improvement, intravenous acetylcysteine should be considered to be administered in patients. It is not recommended to measure the concentration of acetaminophen in the blood to decide on the initiation of the acetylcysteine antidote treatment. The measurement of acetaminophen concentration does not correlate with the degree of hepatic necrosis. Efforts should be made to rule out the possibility of intentional overdose. If it is suspected, a discussion with a toxicologist or poison control center is recommended.

The evolution of almost all causes of acute liver failure should be standardized through specific treatments directed at an underlying etiology. Measures directed against the presumably necroapoptotic process in the liver have no proven efficacy. However, the early application of liver transplant for patients with acetaminophen-induced acute liver failure is the most effective treatment and it can achieve a survival rate of more than 60%. Organ allocation priority time to acute liver failure patients listed for urgent liver transplantation depends on a prognostic system initially based on the King's College Criteria.

Acute liver failure: Specific treatments of underlying causes of acute liver failure

Comprehensive Study on Acute Liver Failure Caused by Acetaminophen Overdose

1. Introduction to Acute Liver Failure

Acute liver failure (ALF) is associated with acetaminophen overdose as a leading cause. ALF is defined as a condition of rapid deterioration of liver function for less than 26 weeks, associated with coagulation disorders (prothrombin time (PT) or International Normalized Ratio (INR) greater than 1.5) and hepatic encephalopathy. Patients may be classified as having a "hyperacute" if it develops within 7 days of the onset of nonspecific coagulopathy, "acute" if it develops between 8 to 28 days, and "subacute" if it develops over 4 weeks. In terms of prognosis, liver transplantation (LTX) is offered to those with hyperacute ALF who have not improved with intensive care medical treatment. Spontaneous survival is more in patients who can be treated medically and do not require LTX. The prognosis of subacute ALF may be better than that of hyperacute ALF. In Europe, ALF occurs at a rate of approximately 3-6 per 1,000,000 individuals per year, with etiology varying according to race, ethnicity, incidence. In our country (Turkey), the incidence of ALF in adults is 1.85 patients per 1,000,000 people each year. It is more common in women than men, with a parity of 3.6:1.

Paracetamol is the most commonly used analgesic and it is also called acetaminophen. Acute liver failure can develop after paracetamol overdose, and it is called paracetamol-induced hepatotoxicity. Acute liver failure can be treated with liver transplantation if it is not treated in the early stage. Acute liver failure can reduce the quality of life, and it can cause death. For those reasons, physicians should identify and begin on a treatment quickly.

1.1. Definition and Classification

Acute liver failure is classified into the following types based on etiology: infectious ALF, ALF associated with toxins, and other factors such as autoimmune diseases. Among them, the most common etiology is drug-induced liver injury (DILI), and paracetamol (acetaminophen) is considered to account for the majority of the cases, especially in Western countries. Acetaminophen is one of the most widely used over-the-counter analgesics and antipyretics, but an overdose can result in acute liver failure.

The definition of acute liver failure is not consistent. In countries with small populations, someone has proposed a clinical disease scoring system to identify ALF; therefore, the term is called: Acute Hepatic Failure (AHF), defined as an acute hepatic injury manifested by a moderate or severe disturbance of synthetic function and encephalopathy in a patient without preexisting liver disease. Typically, there are three criteria to define ALF or its complete phrase Acute Liver Failure (ALF); the ALF is a syndrome whose main features are the rapid development of jaundice, hepatic encephalopathy, and coagulopathy in a patient who did not previously have liver disease. The second one is the time limits for the development of these conditions. The third says that the patient's mental status is absent of other neurologic diseases. In addition, we can add in the description of ALF that it is associated with a high mortality resulting from multiple organ failure in patients with no preexisting liver disease. For now, no standard criteria for the assessment of hepatic encephalopathy in ALF are uniformly accepted. Forton has a clear definition for hepatic encephalopathy in patients with acute liver failure: Mentation grade 1-2 and hepatic encephalopathy (HE) grade 1-2 in a subject without mental status compromise or spinal reflex compromise.

1.2. Epidemiology and Incidence

It is necessary to know right from the start that acetaminophen overdose is the most common cause of ALF in the USA and the majority of the European countries. The overuse of acetaminophen seemed to increase along with biological rhythms of the liver, which made the disease severity 'organic' in the eyes of physicians of traditional East Asian Medicine.

The fact that acute liver failure is considered to be a rare but dramatic and life-threatening event was taken from the term 'fulminant hepatic failure' introduced in 1972. The results of large prospective studies and registries, however, have shown that it occurs in approximately 2.5 cases per 1,000,000 people per year in the UK (n = 120-247), the USA (n = 245-330), and Europe (n = 348-935). The incidence of acetaminophen-induced ALF in the acute liver failure of the above-mentioned registries and studies ranged at 46-54%. It is noteworthy that 40% of 200 cases that resulted in transplantation or death in the later period, i.e. after 3-8 years in the UK Transplant Registry, was attributed to acetaminophen alone. Two U.S. Pediatric Acute Liver Failure Studies Group registries on pediatric ALF showed that acetaminophen was the most common agent of pediatric ALF, accounting for 45 cases (29%) in the 2008 report and 50 (18%) in the 2018 report.

2. Pathophysiology of Acute Liver Failure

2.1. Normal Liver Function

2.2. Mechanism of Acetaminophen Toxicity

3. Clinical Presentation

The main presenting symptoms and signs for the physician appear during the first weeks after the intake of an overdose and are noticed in 50-64% of patients, which are liver tenderness and/or pain, cytolysis, acute-on-chronic liver failure, and super-infection with the progressive occurrence of severe sepsis, septic shock, sepsis-like syndrome, and/or infected ascites. Patients with the best prognosis have minimal symptoms; the groups with intermediate prognosis have full-blown acute liver failure, severe encephalopathy (grade III or IV), and maybe defervescence already at admission; finally, the poorest prognosis group includes severe hyperammonemia (≥ 200 mM/L) and prevalent cerebral edema. Traditionally, hepatic encephalopathy was classified according to the West-Haven criteria, which is based on clinical features. However, these criteria are insufficient, especially for clinical research. While mental status examination and volitional testing are the cornerstone of the clinical work-up and outcome scores, neurophysiological tests such as electroencephalography (EEG), somatosensory evoked potentials (SEPs), brainstem auditory evoked potentials (BAEPs), and magnetic resonance diffusion-weighted images (MRI-DWI) are used as supplementary diagnostic tools. Diagnostic evaluation is directed to the identification of APAP-induced liver injury and the assessment of its severity, thus liver transplant listing.

Acute liver failure is defined as "the rapid development of severe acute liver injury accompanied by hepatic encephalopathy and often failure of other organs" and is a rare and severe condition. The clinical manifestations are diverse over a wide range of patients and are characterized by a progressive loss at the deeper level of altered liver functions leading to severe metabolic, hematological, organ, and hormonal consequences. The first signs perceived by the patients are generally nausea, vomiting, abdominal pain, quickly followed by jaundice and an overall feeling of unwellness.

3.1. Symptoms and Signs

The clinical picture of acute liver failure is dominated by the presence of encephalopathy. The encephalopathy associated with acute liver failure is not different from hepatic encephalopathy of chronic liver failure. The first signs of encephalopathy are insomnia, a feeling of unease, fatigue, and apathy. Confusion states, reduced attention span, impaired concentration, restlessness, and aggressiveness develop in the next stage. At physical examination, the physician may detect belligerence (increased aggressiveness) and delusions. The encephalopathy is accompanied by asterixis and limb rigidity. In severe cases, hepatic coma develops. It manifests with sleepiness, and the patient can be alarmed by giving noxious stimuli. The quadriplegia (decerebrate position) develops, the pupillary reflexes and corneal reflexes are abolished or diminished, and the encephalopathy progresses to coma. In addition, the patient may manifest a sign of cerebral herniation.

3.1. Symptoms and signs. The onset of acute liver encephalopathy is usually more rapid, in less than 24 hours. The clinical manifestations are also much more serious than in acute liver failure. The first signs of hepatic encephalopathy consist of odd behavior, sleepiness, and cognitive changes. In the next stage, the physician may detect a reduced attention span, EEG slowing, photomotor symptoms, and asterixis. In the less severe form of hepatic encephalopathy, the patient could be able to perform arithmetic and writing exercises correctly, whereas in the advanced form, impaired writing but precise reading are common.

3.2. Diagnostic Evaluation

Child Protective Services (CPS) Requests for N-acetylcysteine are frequent and are related to healthcare provider anxiety that they might be "missing" acute hepatic failure, hepatic transaminitis, encephalopathy, or chronic hepatitis. The issue is easily resolved by drawing two liver function tests—a AST and serum bilirubin. ICU CAMS use the following AAP book reference: Guidelines for Acetaminophen Dosing in Infants and Children. In the presence of these dosage guidelines, it is highly unlikely for a parent to exceed the commission's recommendations. Even if a parent had given their child 5 grams, and the dose were repeated just 4-12 hours later, the risk of developing hepatic failure would be present, but minimal: other variables such as the above blood tests, frequency of acetaminophen use, the dose of catecholamines taken, and the time of presentation will also be factors. Finally, if any medication levels are drawn, acetaminophen remains the only drug in America for which there is an anecdotal "antidote": N-acetylcysteine.

Diagnostic evaluation Diagnosis of acute liver failure is determined primarily by history, physical exam and lab testing. Hodges and Salter proposed a probability scale in 1956 which emphasized history and exam as paramount. While this scale is no longer in use, it is important to remember that a few key questions and a good physical are extremely important. In acute liver failure, the coagulation time can be seriously prolonged and any invasive exam (i.e. NG tube placement) should be preceded by transfusing platelets (if less than 40,000), cryoprecipitate, and possibly fresh frozen plasma. In terms of initial laboratory testing, those useful and readily available include: a drug screen, salicylates, acute hepatitis serologies, serologies for acute/chronic viral hepatitis, ammonia and for staff, an acetaminophen level. If the acetaminophen level is negative, the acetaminophen level can be drawn 32 hours post ingestion or 4 hours post last dose of a chronic overdose. If acetaminophen (or if a drug screen was positive or a clinical impression was present), a Salicylate level is the next most important test to be drawn (1/acetylsalicylic acid toxicity is the most common cause of acute hepatic failure after acetaminophen).

Acetaminophen overdose (presenting as either acute single exposures or chronic supratherapeutic ingestion) is the most common cause of acute liver failure in the United States today. Assessing patients presenting with an acute acetaminophen ingestion can be diagnostic if a blood acetaminophen concentration is drawn within 4 to 24 hours of ingestion. In patients presenting more than 24 hours post ingestion, two liver function tests, which many ICUs routinely draw post overdose, are critical for diagnosis of acute liver failure. Finally, while two medication levels are preliminary evidence to seek acetaminaminophen concentrations, an acetaminophen level is the only objective means to "rule out" acetaminophen overdose as a cause for acute hepatic failure. If any of the above criteria are positive for an acetaminophen overdose, the recommended treatment should be N-acetylcysteine (from Mucomyst or a compounding pharmacy using the IV N-acetylcysteine). There are several hospital dosing protocols: a one hour IV preparation or 18.75 hours oral N-acetylcysteine is most efficacious and, if used, there is no need to draw an INHNT or repeat an acetaminophen level. Prosecuting someone for acetaminophen overdose is difficult for many reasons; however, when in doubt, Child Protective Services (CPS) can be notified who can initiate a proper investigation.

4. Management of Acute Liver Failure

The management of acute liver failure includes non-selective inhibition of Kupffer cells, the application of adjuvant antioxidants and other drugs, inhibiting the production of free radicals, preventing lipid peroxidation, anti-cell coherence, liver regeneration, immune regulation, liver transplantation, and extracorporeal liver support therapy. Although studies have shown that corticosteroids and penicillin may be helpful in the treatment of encephalopathy in patients with acute liver failure, they are still uncertain in clinical practice. Due to the rapid progress of acute liver failure and the relatively small time window for liver transplantation, the current main treatment for acute liver failure is liver transplantation, and an early liver transplant is beneficial to the overall prognosis.

According to whether the patients could receive liver transplantation, the management of acute liver failure includes general supportive care and liver transplant. The main treatment includes maintenance of vital functions, prevention of complications, removal of the cause, and drugs. In general, the first priority for patients with acute liver failure is close attention to the airway, breathing, and blood circulation, followed by the management of blood glucose, electrolytes, coagulation, and blood ammonia. Inpatient management of encephalopathy, including the care of critically ill patients, often requires the use of an intensive care unit. In view of the different stages of acute liver failure, the condition of the liver and brain is the key to chronic diseases in treatment.

4.1. General Supportive Care

Management of acetaminophen overdose: N-Acetylcysteine (NAC) reduces mortality with early acute liver failure due to acetaminophen overdose, regardless of plasma acetaminophen levels. For everyone who presents ingestions with: plasma acetaminophen above the "possible toxicity line" of the "200-line" nomograph, 10 mcg/mL at 4 hours or 4 mcg/mL at any time after 10 hours, obtain a 4 o'clock specimen and discuss management with an inpatient. D-dimer levels can be elevated in patients with acetaminophen hepatotoxicity. The use of D-dimer levels in regard to PT as predictors of poor outcomes could be of value in these patients and is worth further study in a large database. Plasma lipids should be monitored, given the possibility of hepatic dysfunction in the background. Anaerobic metabolism results in lactate production and, consequently, lactic acidosis. Unlike most other forms of metabolic acidosis, the presence of lactic acidosis does not always predict a poor outcome. Urea and both creatinine and urea increase in ALF: unlike the kidney, the liver contains high levels of both creatinine and urea in hepatocytes. When the liver is damaged, both creatinine and urea are released from damaged hepatocytes and the levels increase in the plasma. Needling and measuring a catheter with respect to intra-abdominal pressure is the first step in the diagnosis. If pressure exceeds 12, the patient is at risk for hepatic dysfunction in the background.

General supportive care: The goals can be regarded as hemodynamic monitoring, with management largely dependent on the degree of hemodynamic instability, and can include fluid resuscitation, vasopressors, and intubation with sedation and neuromuscular blockade. Some patients with marked hypoperfusion may benefit from an intra-arterial catheter to measure the cardiac index, pulmonary artery catheterization to monitor filling pressures, or central venous catheterization for CVP monitoring. Patients require neurologic examination for the detection of herniation as a potential cause for altered mental status. Patients with clinical signs of elevated ICP, such as hypertension, bradycardia, and abnormal posturing, are generally given a 250 cc 3% hypertonic saline bolus, in an attempt to reduce raised ICP and to prevent progression to brainstem herniation. Blood glucose and serum electrolyte levels should also be evaluated and kept within normal limits. Chest radiography is appropriate for identifying aspiration, pulmonary edema, and pneumonia. ECG should be used to rule out any cardiac ischemia and as a baseline for QTc interval, which should be periodically monitored. International normalized ratio (INR), partial thromboplastin time (PTT), and fibrinogen, serum electrolytes, BUN, and creatinine, and arterial blood gas should also be monitored. In all, the management of ALF is dubious; as the cause and pathophysiology vary according to the etiology, it is difficult to have a consensus in the guidelines regarding the biochemical treatments of ALF.

4.2. Specific Treatment Options

Antioxidants can reduce oxidative stress, such as N-acetyl-cysteine (NAC), but evidence is still limited. Liver transplantation can be performed after liver support systems, blood clotting parameters (including INR), brain function, hemodynamic, and infection regulation. Liver transplantation is done when there is no hope of being cured. The 21-day period is when the liver transplant is performed. The optimal timing of liver transplantation is within 10 days, but if possible, liver transplantation should be performed after the patient's COMP score reaches 9.

Acetaminophen overdose For acetaminophen overdose, there is a treatment protocol known as the Rumack-Matthew nomogram. Giving acetylcysteine pills and injections within 8-10 hours of overdose reduced the number of patients with acute liver failure. In patients with acetaminophen overdose, acetylcysteine is administered at a dose of 150 mg/kg for 15-30 minutes, then 50 mg/kg for 4 hours, and the prescription can last up to 72 hours. However, adverse reactions such as rashes and anaphylaxis can occur with acetylcysteine. For acute liver failure patients with stage 1 and INR > 2.3 and/or bilirubin < 23 mg/dl, cynarin is combined with antiviral agents such as tenofovir and adefovir.

Acute liver failure Acute liver failure does not have specific treatment modalities. Usually, the treatment is conservative supportive care. In conservative care, specific treatment options are limited. Some options can be presented from. One option is the use of a drug called acetylcysteine, which removes acetaminophen-related toxins from the liver. In some patients with acute liver failure, liver transplantation can be performed. The role of liver transplantation and when it should be performed is established by a liver transplant center.

5. Prognosis and Complications

5.1. Factors Affecting Prognosis

5.2. Potential Complications

6. Prevention Strategies

Public health interventions are outside the scope of this review, but they have been shown to have a large level of effectiveness in the field of ALF, following their implementation in the UK in 1998. Small pilot studies have demonstrated high feasibility of bioethics review and consent for the study of a vulnerable population, and the informed consent process is recommended for ethically designing such human subject studies. Future population-based studies may examine multiple approaches taken at multiple levels, including preclinical development of antidotal therapy and public health policy interventions.

Preventive strategies in reducing the incidence of acetaminophen-related ALF include public health intervention such as regulatory and legislative action, labeling, education and professional training, and other interventions aiming to decrease the occurrence of drug overdose. Specifically, regulatory measures have been proposed that would lower the toxic as well as the maximum tolerated daily single dose; legislative action proposes to restrict the availability, for example, with regards to distributing the drug without prescription; label changes typically take into account the first two days of overdose and include measures aiming to reduce further self-harm; generic warnings include discouraging physicians from prescribing acetaminophen in high doses or in combination with other products. Patient education entails efforts to reduce the likelihood of unintentional overdose, for example, by counseling against prescription of other products with acetaminophen, and to encourage early presentation to the healthcare system. Finally, continuous education of nurses and pharmacists, as well as emergency medicine personnel, is expected to contribute to reducing overdose incidence as well as improving the delivery of care in Western countries.

6.1. Public Health Interventions

There are also background public health approaches, whose efficacy is not well studied. These include providing analgesics for small numbers of tablets at no increased expense or inconvenience of purchase, thereby decreasing the sizes of stockpiles in the community, or actively recommending N-acetylcysteine to definitively classify ALF patients, and thereby provide a disincentive for certain attempts at suicide. Finally, decreasing current suicidogenic environmental variables may unsuccessfully fuel an individual's latent suicidal ideation such that when the environment becomes less favorable, as studied by Caine in the context of charismatic leadership in certain religious denominations, the proportion of individuals who act upon their suicidal ideation to actually commit suicide may paradoxically increase.

The second category focuses on the public health interventions that have been instituted to prevent ALF. Despite a rather consistent rate of acetaminophen overdose over the last several decades, the incidence of DILI related to acetaminophen has not changed markedly. This finding suggests that prevention may proceed along two lines: preventing overdose and preventing toxicity after overdose has occurred. Prevention of overdose is similar to that of prevention of suicide and includes strategies at multiple socioecologic levels. Deterrence involves criminalization and education emailed to the potentially offending group. Active practice of ongoing counseling about limitation of product quantity per container may deter individuals from purchasing.

For individual patients, the subject of acetaminophen overdose prevention is a public choice that requires physicians to provide information about it. Educating people about acetaminophen and overdose is significant. The presentation should emphasize the benefits and dosage as the main factors. Education's motivation is to disseminate details regarding treatment ingestion and the concept or potential impact of poisoning. Acetaminophen is the product that should take center stage or be included specifically. Knowledge of acetaminophen is a basic part of this token disorder. This article, along with related literature, highlights the main features that experts should investigate. A brief introduction is given to show the importance of the topic. For clarity, a brief explanation is given in sections 4 and 6 when certain details are presented. Subsequently, more specific aspects related to the given topic were presented. Query response inclusion criteria used to determine the relevance of queries. Exclude references and comments in the last step.

With acetaminophen overdose being the predominant cause of acute liver failure, both preventively and involuntarily, several reports, programs, and campaigns advocate patient education. This concept also reflects our opinion that patient education and knowledge reduction can support affected individuals in making informed decisions about their health and taking measures to minimize the incidence of acute liver failure. Without the patient's informed approval, do not advise the treatment.

These prevention programs are too wide and exist to show working protective interventions at the population level.

7. Conclusion and Future Directions

Future research directions include the incorporation of risk of liver failure scores, which are already in use when predicting the likelihood of spontaneous survival when listed for OLT with paracetamol-induced acute liver failure, with those to help in the prediction of an initial assessment of social service requirement. Cost-of-illness studies are underway to extrapolate the economics of patients presenting in the emergency department and those admitted into the hospital with a paracetamol overdose at risk of liver failure compared to the non-paracetamol overdose requiring NAC in the USA. Significant heterogeneity exists worldwide in the reports of long-term damage after acetaminophen-induced acute liver injury. The association with underlying liver disease is not clear, and it has been suggested that some patients may experience a chronic reduction in liver function and may eventually require transplant up to 5.5 years later. Further collaborations are underway to jointly report the epidemiology of and post-acute liver injury from acetaminophen.

Data from close to 3,300 patients have been collated, over a quarter of these from the United States' ALFSG, providing a comprehensive in-depth study of this high-impact condition. Although centered predominantly on the cause of acetaminophen and unintentional/undesired overdose, it is clear that there is a cohort of patients who are 'at-risk' of taking further overdoses, some of whom go on to develop liver failure. Analyses of the studied cohort show that those who have taken multiple overdoses have more progressive liver injury, are more likely to go to OLT, and have worsened outcome (53.8% 2-week mortality versus an already poor 36.7%). However, despite controlling for the important factor of time since overdose, six more clinically discriminatory dynamic 'at-risk of developing liver failure' indices were developed that must be tested in other datasets. Physical health (blood pressure, respiratory rate, creatinine, INR, lactate, and pH) was found to more accurately predict the need for an OLT than blood biochemistry.

www.ingramcontent.com/pod-product-compliance
Lightning Source LLC
Chambersburg PA
CBHW070801250726
48662CB00004B/1925

* 9 7 9 8 3 3 4 6 1 0 5 7 6 *